Diabetic Diet Plan

The beginners guide to healthy eating & Keeping the Flavor!

By

Kay Hersom

Five Star Reviews!

*"**Amazing Resource** -I loved this book! The recipes and suggestions for healthy eating are superb! Everyone could benefit from the information contained here. I would definitely recommend this to anyone wanting to improve their health, as well as diabetics. You can even eat dessert!"*

*"**Great Food Guide for Diabetics** - As a sufferer of Type 2 diabetes, I'm always on the lookout for sources of good information about managing my diet and lifestyle. Kay Herson has written a smart, basic food guide for diabetics with a helpful food plan. Even better, she includes 18 recipes for breakfast meals, appetizers, lunch and dinner suggestions and even desserts. I'm cooking my first one today!"*

*"**Love the Recipes** - My husband has type 2 diabetes and he loves to eat. He was raised much like the authors Mom was and food is a comfort to him. Well it's up to me to provide tasty and healthy food for him. With these recipes and plan he will not feel deprived and not even know he's eating healthy food. The recipes and pictures made me hungry. Great job."*

Diabetic Diet Plan: The beginners guide to healthy eating

& Keeping the Flavor!

By Kay Hersom

First Published, 2013 Printed in the United States of America

Hersom House Publishing

3365 NE 45th St. Suite 101

Ocala, Florida 34479

This eBook is intentionally published on the Amazon Kindle platform so that you can enjoy it in quick snippets on any mobile device, while in the grocery store, or planning a meal. A Kindle eReader device is not required to enjoy this book; simply download the Kindle App to any Smartphone or mobile device you own to enjoy your Kindle library on the go!

Notice

This book is intended as a reference volume only, not as a medical manual. The information given here is designed to help you make informed decisions about your health. It is not intended as a substitute for any treatment that may have been prescribed by your doctor. If you suspect that you have a medical problem, I urge you to seek competent medical help. As when starting any exercise or diet program consult your doctor before beginning.

Introduction

My career exposes me to many individuals who have multiple medical issues relating to diabetes. Unfortunately, poor eating habits and mismanaging glucose (blood sugar) levels may have contributed to their poor health. Heart disease, loss of limbs, poor eye-sight or blindness, and kidney failure that requires dialysis, is common.

A year and one half ago my mother was diagnosed with type 2 diabetes. My family immediately envisioned the worst as far as her future health. We knew a change in her eating habits would need to improve so my family committed to helping her with a lifestyle change.

My mother, as bright and intelligent as she was at 67 years of age, (sorry Momma) had never in her life owned a cell phone or ever operated a computer, let alone own one. So when she asked me for a little help in finding some new diabetic recipes that actually would taste good and have some flavor, and not taste like cardboard like the doctor's pamphlet recipes, I agreed.

Momma was raised in rural America where carbs and sugars were part of the staples of life. A common meal was meat (usually fried) and potatoes covered with lots of gravy, biscuits or cornbread lathered with butter, sweet tea, and dessert after every meal. And evidently, vegetables were not tasty enough naturally because equal parts of bacon or some kind of pork fat was always added.

I could see the frustration she was experiencing. She lost weight due partly to eating a balanced diet, and in part to not eating much at all because everything tasting so bland. I needed to find a starting point for her, to equip her with some basic tools that would define which foods to seek out and which ones to run from, how to meal plan to meet her nutritional needs, and feel as though she was able to make Daddy happy. And, what could she order when Daddy took her out to eat?

Ironically, at that time my younger sister was dealing with gestational diabetes during her pregnancy so she volunteered to come over and "taste test" the new recipes I created, she's always been helpful that way. After hours of researching the Internet gathering data and ideas, and trying recipes... I put together this guide to help Momma and others get started with their diabetic diet plan without giving up the delicious flavors of food... only the frustration.

So You're Diabetic

If you are reading these words, most likely you or someone you know and love has diabetes. In the U. S. slightly over 7 percent of people, which is estimated to be around 19 million, have diabetes. The disease of diabetes occurs when the body does not produce or properly use a hormone called insulin, which is needed to transform sugar, starches and other food into energy for our bodies. The cause of diabetes is still unknown. However genetics and environmental factors such as being overweight and lack of exercise appear to play a big part. So your lifestyle and what you put in your body directly affects your health, and more specifically your diabetes.

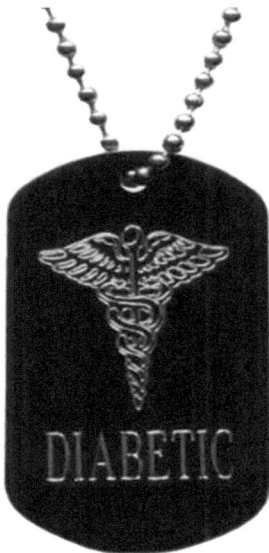

Type What?

There are three types of diabetes. Type 1, Type 2 and Gestational.

Type 1

This is when the pancreas stops producing insulin. Insulin lets blood sugar or glucose enter into the body's cells to be used for energy. With no insulin the body's cells can't get the glucose they need and too much sugar builds up in the blood system.

Type 2

This condition occurs when insulin is either less produced, or is not absorbed properly by the body. In either case, the body absorbs less insulin required to keep the rising blood sugar in control. Losing weight can help control blood glucose. Weight loss can offer other health benefits too, such as lowering high blood pressure, lowering your risk of heart disease, and relieving joint pain.

Gestational

Gestational only occurs during pregnancy from a result of to much hormone production in the body. This temporary form of insulin opposition generally goes away after giving birth, but females who have experienced this are at risk for later developing diabetes.

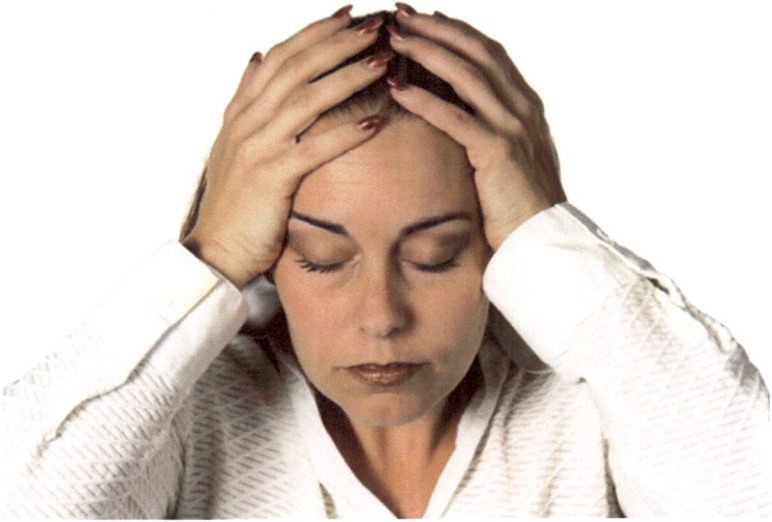

How to Plan the Diabetic Diet Plan

As frustrating as it may feel, relax, it's not as complicated as you may think. Information is power but rule # 1, don't over think it.

A diabetic diet plan, medically known as medical nutrition therapy (MNT), involves eating a mixture of highly nutritious foods in moderate amounts, during the regular meal times. This is not a restrictive diet; it is a healthy eating plan that is rich in nutrients, low in calories and fats and emphasizing on vegetables, fruits and whole grains. Almost everyone would benefit from eating on this type of plan because it helps control the amount of blood sugar levels and keeps the weight off. Maintaining a safe range of blood sugar level is the key objective for a diabetic, so make healthy food choices and keep track of what you eat.

Recommended healthy and nutritious diabetic diet foods:

Healthy Carbohydrates

During digestion, simple carbohydrates such as sugars and complex carbohydrates such as starches break down into blood glucose. It is important to have healthy carbohydrates like fruits, vegetables, whole grains, legumes and low-fat dairy products. Like the saying goes, "An apple (with skin on) a day keeps the doctor away."

Foods Rich in Fiber

All parts of plant foods, that your body can't digest or absorb, are high in fiber. As stated above, it is important to include vegetables, fruits, whole grains and lentils. Other foods include walnuts, almonds, brown rice, oatmeal, whole-wheat flour and wheat bran. Dark green vegetables such as spinach, kale, broccoli, and romaine lettuce are rich in fiber and are most beneficial when eaten raw. Consuming black beans is not only rich in fiber and protein; they contain magnesium, folate, and antioxidants. Incorporating fiber into your snacks and meals will help to control blood sugar levels and can also decrease the risk of heart disease.

Heart-healthy Fish

Fish contains healthy fats like omega-3 fatty acids, a polyunsaturated fat, which reduces the chances of experiencing cardiovascular disease. It also helps reduce blood pressure and inflammation. Fish can be a good alternative to high-fat meats. Cold water fish are the best, like salmon, halibut, tuna and herring. Other foods to include in your daily plan that are rich in this nutrient are flack seeds (ground), soybeans, sardines, and tofu.

Good Fats

Eating foods containing monounsaturated and polyunsaturated fats such as avocados, olives, canola and peanut oils, and nuts like almonds, pecans, and walnuts can help lower your cholesterol levels. However, eat them in moderate amounts as all fats are high in calories.

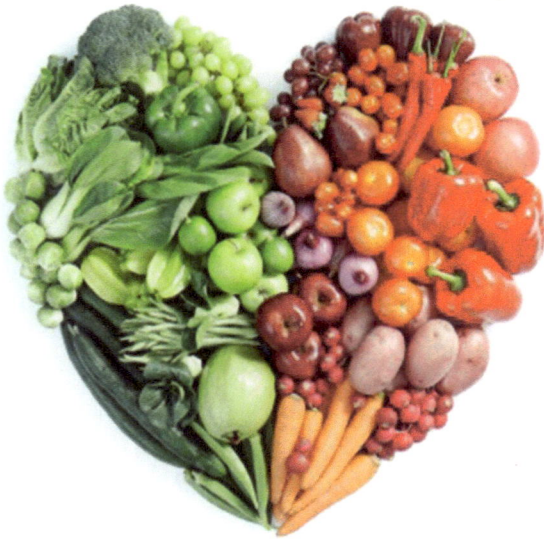

Foods to Avoid

The potential of heart disease and stroke because of clogged and hardened arteries from diabetes is a risk. So you need to know that foods containing the following can work against your heart healthy goal.

Avoid foods that are high in fat. Saturated fats and trans-fats should be reduced or even eliminated from your diet. These fats increase the level of your LDL or bad cholesterol, which increases the triglyceride levels in your blood. High triglyceride levels are bad for your heart because they immediately increase after you eat, which can cause high blood pressure, lead to plaque buildup in your arteries, and atherosclerosis, a condition that can limit blood flow to your brain, heart and other parts of your body.

Foods that come from animals such as butter, milk, cheese, meat, among others, have saturated fats. Some plant based foods also contain this fat, like coconut, coconut oil, palm oil and cocoa butter. Trans- fat is the most dangerous fat for your heart. Avoid trans-fats as much as possible since they increase your bad cholesterol and lower your good cholesterol. Some of the common sources of cholesterol include the high fat animal proteins such as egg yolks, liver, shellfish and high fat dairy products. Foods like, margarine, shortening, packaged and some frozen foods, baked goods, chips, crackers, even some soups, contain trans-fats. Aim for less than 2,300 milligrams of sodium a day. Look for low sodium foods and use sodium substitutes.

Keeping your blood sugar levels under control cannot be stressed enough, if your level runs too high it can cause serious chronic problems like kidney and heart damage.

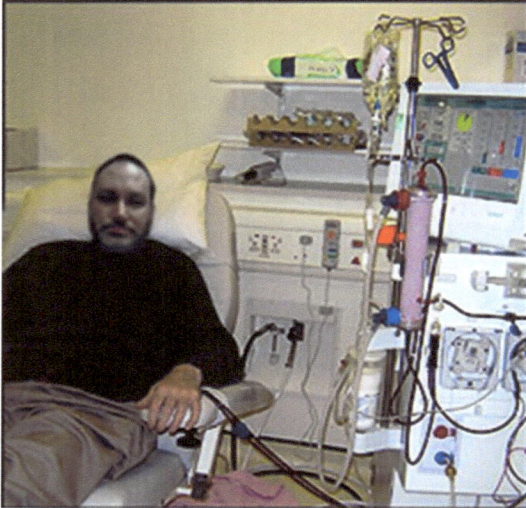

Mr. J. Howard – Kidney Dialysis

Once you know the foods to eat and the foods to avoid, you now have to know that you should also control the portion of your food. A helpful tool may be to purchase smaller plates and refrain from going back for seconds.

Grocery Shopping Helper

The following is a list I put together to help me during the visits to the grocery store. This is by no means a full or compressive list but simply a guide and reminder of what foods I should be thinking of when planning our meals.

Produce

- Fresh Fruit - the more variety the better, mix up the colors

- Fresh Fruit - the more variety the better, mix up the colors

Fish –Frozen and/or Fresh

- Non-breaded fillets

- Non-breaded shellfish

Meats

- Turkey

- Turkey Bacon

- Turkey Sausage

- Lean low-sodium turkey or chicken sandwich meat

- Skinless chicken

- Lean cuts of beef

- Lean hamburger 90/10

Canned & Dried Food

- Fruits canned in juice, not in syrup

- Vegetables low-sodium, and fat-free when available

- Soups low sodium, low-fat

- Canned chicken, low-sodium

- Canned fish, tuna and/or salmon

- Whole grain breakfast cereal

- Oatmeal

- Whole wheat pasta

- Brown rice

- Wild rice

- Whole wheat and whole grain breads

- Whole wheat flour

- Pasta sauce

- Peanut Butter

- Olive Oil

- Canola Oil

- Balsamic Vinegar

- Cooking Sprays

- Salt substitute

Snacks

- Nuts - peanuts, almonds, etc

- Dried fruit - raisins, dates, cranberries, etc

- Popcorn low sodium, low-fat (light)

- Baked potato chips low-sodium

- Seeds, sunflower or flax

- Whole wheat/grain crackers low-sodium

The Exchange System

A recommended approach to mastering your diabetic meal plan may be to use the "exchange system". This trading system groups foods into categories such as carbohydrates, meats and meat substitutes, and fats.

With the system you may trade one serving of food group with another serving of food group because the effect on your blood sugar level is about the same. For instance, you may want to eat a pasta serving instead of a meat serving for lunch.

Glycemic Index

Another way to help manage your diabetes is to use the glycemic index to select foods, especially carbohydrates. Foods linked to higher increases in blood sugar have a greater glycemic index. To minimize increased levels of glucose, choose foods that have a low glycemic index. Complex carbohydrates that are high in fiber, such as whole grain rice, breads or cereals, have a lower glycemic index compared to simple carbohydrates such as white bread or white rice. Keep in mind that not all low index foods are healthy. Some foods that have lower glycemic index values are high in fat.

Read the Label

First thing to learn is READ the LABEL. Do not just assume something is good for you just because it says all natural, organic or low fat. When shopping with my mother we found all kinds of things that were good for her in one area, but bad for her in another. For instance, a jar of pasta sauce labeled "all natural ingredients", but having through the roof sodium levels. Always check food labels for carbohydrates and sugars because many high-fiber foods have sugar added to increase their taste.

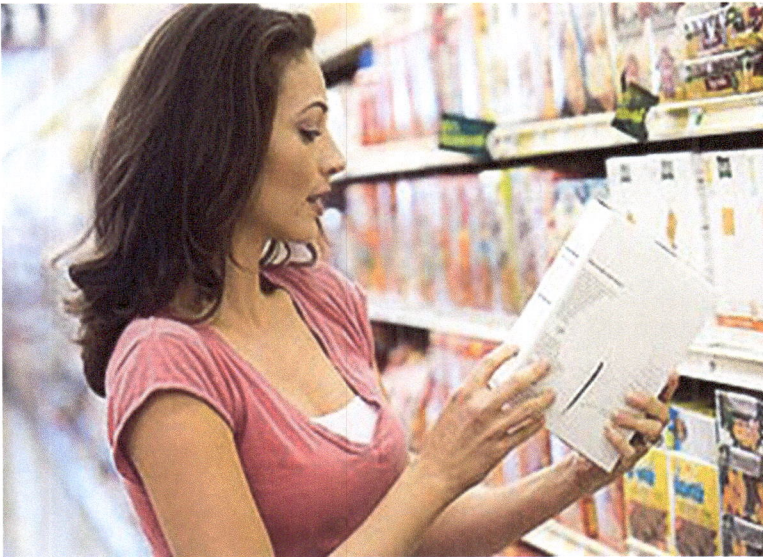

Sample Meal Plans for Beginners

Your size and physical activity level should be taken into account when determining your daily meal plan. A sample menu below is based on a person with diabetes who needs 1,200 to 1,600 calories a day.

> Breakfast: Whole-wheat toast, one piece of fruit and 6 ounces of non-fat Greek yogurt.

> Lunch: Cheese and veggie whole grain pita, medium apple with 2 tablespoons of almond butter.

> Dinner: Beef stroganoff; 1/2 cup of carrots; side salad with 1 ½ cups of spinach, 1/2 of a tomato, 1/4 cup of chopped bell pepper, 2 teaspoons olive oil, 1 1/2 teaspoons of red wine vinegar.

> Snacks: Two unsalted rice cakes topped with 1 ounce of light spreadable cheese or one orange with 1/2 cup of 1% low-fat cottage cheese.

Avoid Sweets? No not really as long as you use the exchange system. Of course this needs to be done in moderation, but a little treat is ok every now and then. If you have a craving for some chocolate or pie just remember to keep the portion size small. Then substitute it for another starchy carb you might eat on your daily plan, like a potato or a piece of bread.

Here is a daily sample of a heart healthy menu:

> Breakfast: One cup of oatmeal flavored with cinnamon and raisins, along with a cup of coffee.

> Lunch: Low-sodium turkey and tomato sandwich on wheat bread, two cups of fresh spinach leafed salad sprinkled with almonds, and a glass of skim milk.

> Dinner: Grilled salmon with brown rice, steamed broccoli and cauliflower on the side, and a glass of iced tea or red wine.

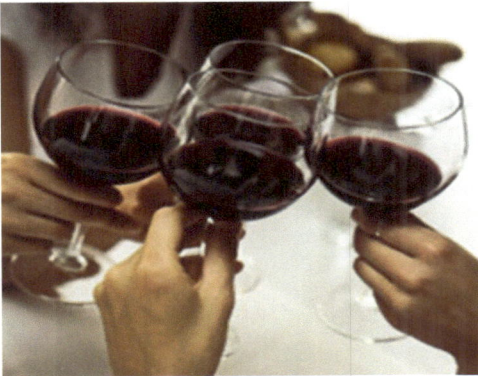

Though changing your eating habits can be challenging at first, once you get used to your daily meal plan, your body will love you! Cheers to you and healthy new lifestyle!!

God Bless,

Kay Hersom

Keeping the Flavor!

Day Starters

Whole Wheat Waffles Topped with Berries and Yogurt

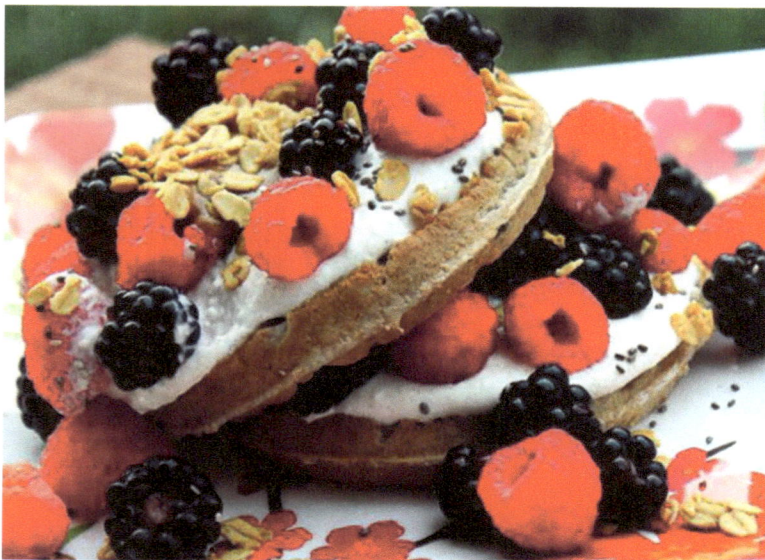

Whole Wheat Waffles Topped with Berries and Yogurt

Ingredients:

- 1 1/2 cups Premium Whole Wheat Flour

- 2 teaspoons baking powder

- 1/2 teaspoon salt

- 2 tablespoons sugar

- 2 egg whites

- 1 large egg or egg substitute

- 1 teaspoon vanilla extract

- 1 1/2 cups lukewarm milk

- 1/3 cup melted butter or canola oil

- Berries of choice, strawberries, blueberries, blackberries and raspberries

- 3 tablespoons of vanilla yogurt – low fat

- 2 tablespoons of granola mix

Preparation

Preheat your waffle iron while you make the waffle batter. Mix together the flour, baking powder, salt, and sugar. In a separate bowl, mix together the egg, milk, and butter or oil. Take whites and beat in a bowl with a mixer until fluffy.

Mix together the wet and dry ingredients, stirring just until combined. Then fold in egg whites, the batter will be a bit lumpy. Cook the waffles until golden.

To serve, top with yogurt, berries and/or granola. Makes approximately 3 Belgian-style waffles.

El Rancho Breakfast Burritos

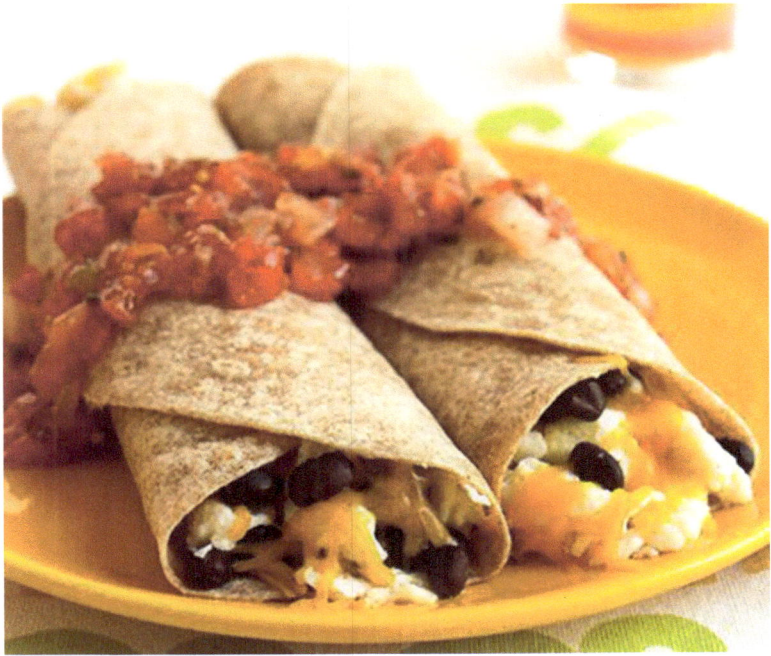

El Rancho Breakfast Burritos

Ingredients:

- 2 eggs or egg substitute

- 2 whole wheat tortillas

- 1 cup fat free cheese Mexican blend

- ¼ cup canned black beans, rinsed

- 1 Roma tomato, chopped

- ¼ cup onion, chopped

- Fresh Cilantro sprigs

- 2 tablespoons fat free sour cream

- Salsa for topping

Preparation

Cover the bottom of a medium sized frying pan with cooking spray. Scramble the egg substitute until cooked. Place the scrambled eggs on the tortillas. Sprinkle with cheese and then lay the black beans over the cheese and eggs. Cover with chopped tomato and onion, then add 1 tablespoon of sour cream to each tortilla. Add fresh cilantro to taste.

Roll each tortilla into a wrap and microwave for 30 seconds to melt cheese. Then plate and top with desired amount of salsa.

French Toast Stuffed with Strawberries and Cheese

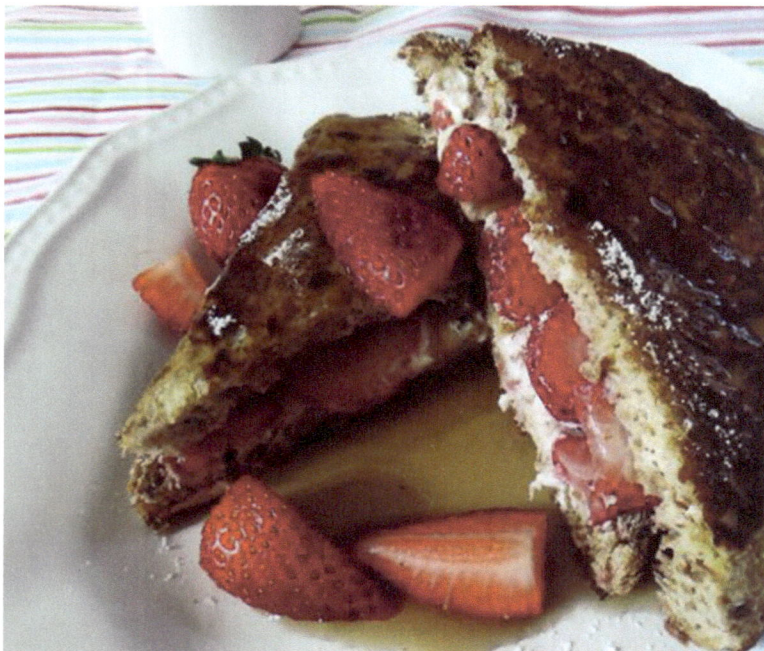

French Toast Stuffed with Strawberries and Cheese

Ingredients:

- 2 slices wheat bread

- 6 strawberries, sliced

- 1/2 oz cream cheese, fat free or flavored Greek yogurt

- 1 egg white or egg substitute

- 1 teaspoon strawberry jam, sugar free

- 1 packet of artificial sweetener

- 1 tablespoons low fat milk

- 1/4 tsp vanilla extract

Preparation

In a bowl, add egg, milk, vanilla extract, and sweetener. Mix and set aside. In another bowl add strawberry jam, cream cheese (or yogurt) and mix together.

On one slice of bread add your cream cheese mixture and top with strawberry slices. Add other slice of bread to the top.

Carefully dip your stuffed bread into the egg mixture; carefully turn over to cover the other side with the egg mixture. Place in a skillet and cook until bottom is lightly brown, and carefully flip and cook until bottom is lightly brown. To serve cut diagonal, top with strawberries and sugar free maple syrup. Enjoy!

Savory Appetizers

Black Bean Dip

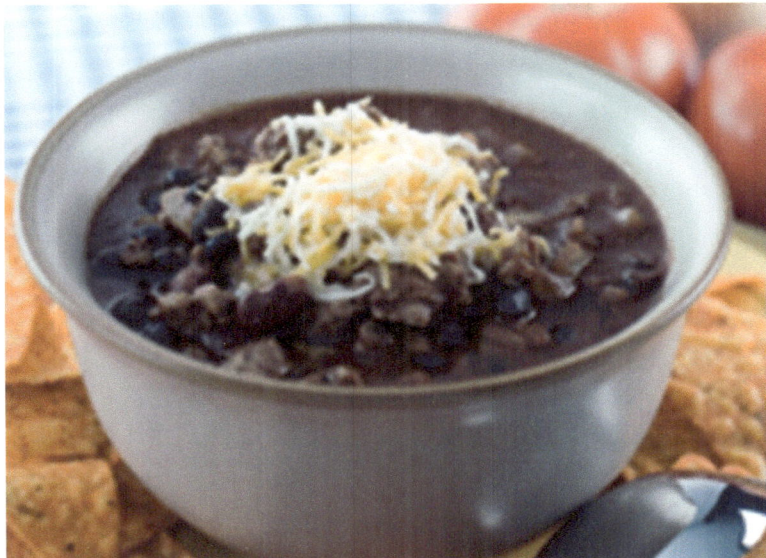

Black Bean Dip

Ingredients:

- 1 can of refried black beans (fat free)

- 1 tablespoon minced garlic

- 2 tablespoons olive oil

- ½ teaspoon ground cumin

- ½ teaspoon cayenne pepper (optional)

- 1 teaspoon lime juice

- ¼ cup grated cheddar cheese

Preparation

In a blender or food processor, mix all the ingredients except the cheese and blend until smooth. Sprinkle grated cheese on top of the dip when serving. Serve with your favorite tortilla chips, crackers, or pita triangles. May be served at room temperature or warmed up.

Provolone Topped Portobello with Balsamic Vinegar

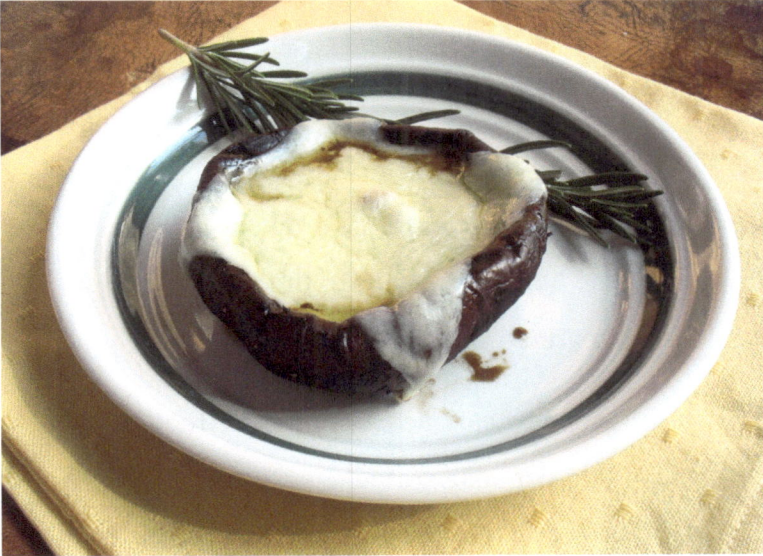

Provolone Topped Portobello with Balsamic Vinegar

Ingredients:

- 4 Portobello mushrooms cleaned and de-stemmed

- 1/2 cup balsamic vinegar

- 1 tablespoon brown sugar or 1 packet of artificial sweetener

- 1/8 teaspoon dried rosemary

- 1 teaspoon minced garlic

- 1/4 cup grated provolone cheese

Preparation

Preheat the oven broiler to 425 degrees. Coat a glass baking dish with cooking spray. Place the mushrooms in the dish bottom side up.

In a bowl mix the vinegar, brown sugar or artificial sweetener, rosemary and garlic. Add mushrooms to the mixture and set aside for 10 minutes to marinate.

Broil the mushrooms, turning once, until they're tender, about 4 minutes on each side. Sprinkle grated cheese over each mushroom and continue to broil until the cheese melts. Serve immediately.

Flavorful Meals

Grilled Shrimp and Mango Salad

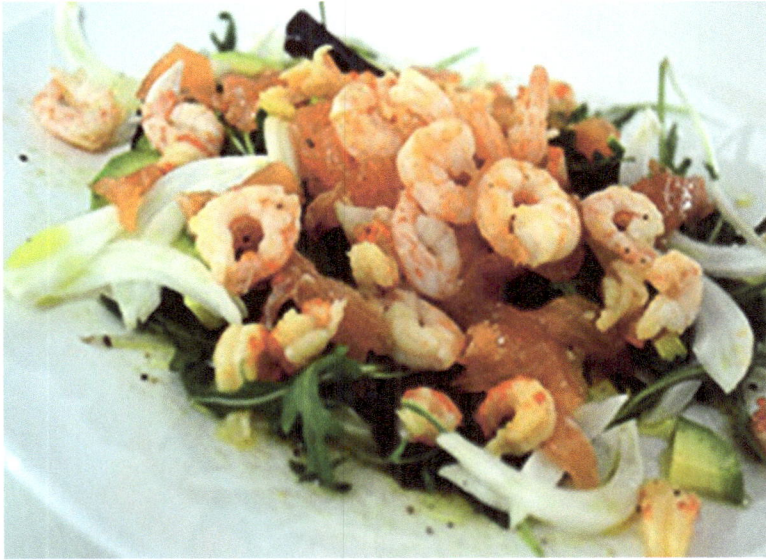

Grilled Shrimp and Mango Salad

Ingredients:

- 2 mangoes, peeled and shredded

- 2 green onions thinly sliced

- 1/3 cup lime juice

- 2 tablespoons fish sauce, or use low sodium soy sauce

- 1 teaspoon sugar

- 1 tablespoon of fresh minced garlic

- 1 serrano pepper, seeded, minced

- 1 pound medium shrimp

- 2 cups salad greens

- lime slices, for garnish

Preparation

Mix green onions, lime juice, fish sauce, sugar, garlic, and pepper in a bowl. Combine shredded mango. Chill while preparing shrimp.

Shell and devein shrimp and divide into 4 portions. Thread each portion onto a slender metal skewer. Grill shrimp on a medium hot grill, covered, for about 3 minutes on each side, or until opaque but still a bit moist in the center of thickest parts.

Place salad greens on a platter; mound mango mixture onto the greens using a slotted spoon. Slide shrimp off skewers and place over the mango salad and garnish with lime slices.

Serves 4

Chicken or Turkey Chili with White Beans

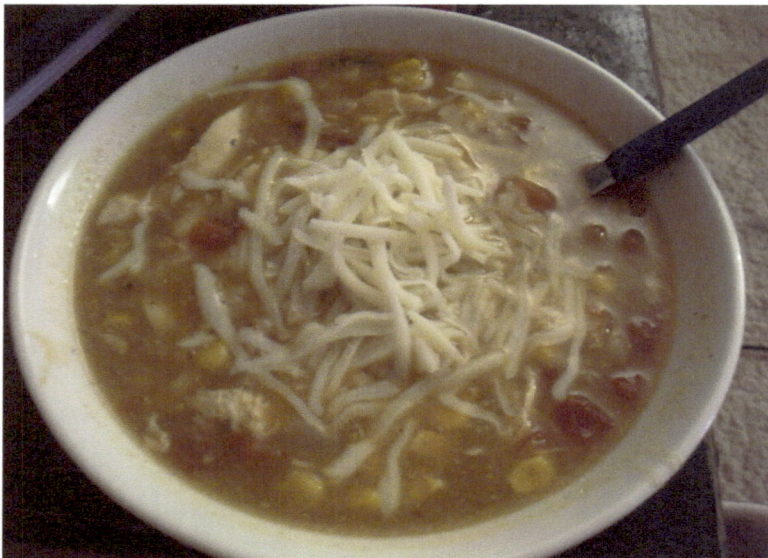

Chicken or Turkey Chili with White Beans

Ingredients:

- 2 tablespoons canola oil

- 1 medium onion chopped

- 2 tablespoons fresh minced garlic

- 2 cans Cannellini beans also known as white kidney

- 1 can chicken broth, low-sodium & fat-free 14.5 oz

- 1 can tomatillos drained and chopped 18oz

- 1 can diced tomatoes 16oz

- 1 can sweet corn 16oz

- 1 can diced green chilies 7oz

- ½ teaspoon dried oregano

- ½ teaspoon ground coriander

- ¼ teaspoon ground cumin

- ¼ teaspoon cayenne pepper (optional)

- 1 pound chicken or turkey diced and cooked

- Salt & pepper to taste

Preparation

Heat oil in soup pan, then sauté garlic and onion until soft.

Mix in broth, tomatoes, chilies, tomatillos and spices. Then bring to a boil.

Simmer for 10 minutes.

Mix in beans, corn and meat, season with salt and pepper to taste and simmer for 5 additional minutes.

Sesame Chicken on a Stick with Peanut Sauce

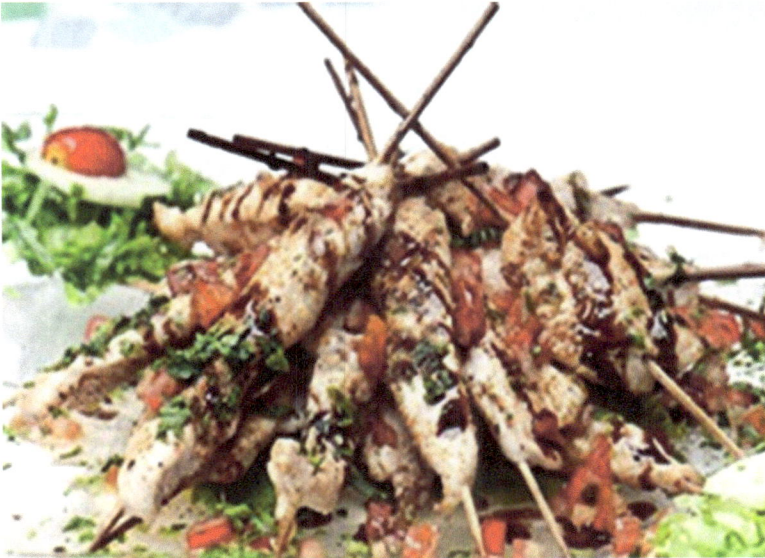

Sesame Chicken on a Stick with Peanut Sauce

Ingredients:

- 1/3 cup low sodium soy sauce

- 2 tablespoons honey

- 1 tablespoon sesame oil

- 6 sliced green onions

- 1 red bell pepper, chopped into 1 inch chunks

- 3 boneless skinless chicken breast cut into 1 inch strips

- 12 bamboo skewers, soaked in for water for 1 hour

- 3 tablespoons sesame seeds

- 1 bag shredded lettuce

Peanut Sauce

- 1 c. low sodium low fat chicken broth

- 1/4 c. shelled, skinned fresh roasted peanuts

- 1 tbsp. fresh lemon juice

- 1 tbsp. minced fresh ginger

- 1/4 tsp. chili powder

- 1 garlic clove, minced

- Salt

Preparation

In a large bowl combine soy sauce, honey, sesame oil, green onions, and red pepper and stir well. Slice the chicken breast lengthwise into 1/4 inch thick pieces. Skewer the chicken slices and place into a zip lock bag. Pour the marinade into the bag and place in refrigerator for at least one hour. Make peanut sauce. Remove the chicken skewers from zip lock bag and set aside. Sprinkle the sesame seeds over the chicken and preheat grill.

In a sauce pan pour remaining marinade and cook over a medium heat until liquid is reduced to the consistency of a sauce, turn temperature down to lowest setting. Place chicken skewers on the grill at medium fire for four minutes per side, until cooked through.

To serve, garnish platter with lettuce, then stack skewers and then pour reduced marinade over chicken skewers. Enjoy!

Peanut Sauce

For peanut sauce: Mix first 6 ingredients in blender until smooth, about 1 minute. Transfer to saucepan. Simmer until thick enough to coat spoon, stirring constantly, about 10 minutes. Pinch of salt to taste.

Vegetable Lasagna

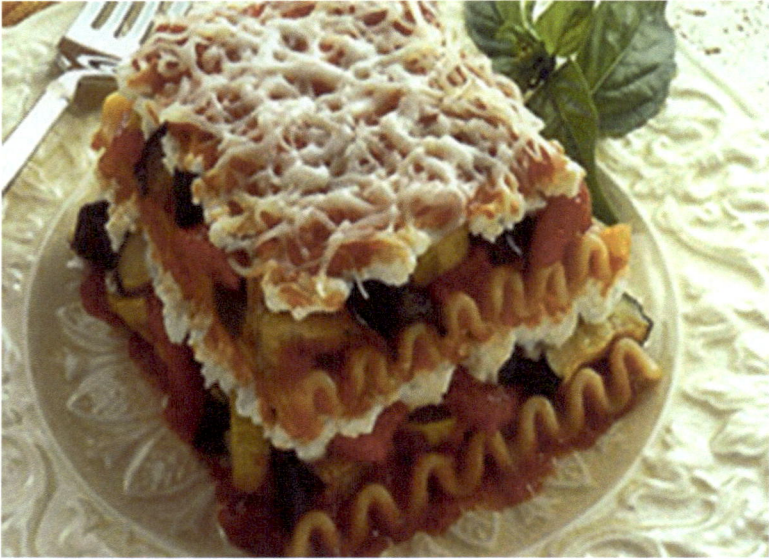

Vegetable Lasagna

Ingredients:

- 2 yellow squash, halved lengthwise and thinly sliced
- 4 medium zucchini, halved lengthwise and thinly sliced
- 1 (8-oz.) package sliced fresh mushrooms
- 1 tablespoon garlic, minced
- Vegetable cooking spray
- 1 medium-size red bell pepper, chopped
- 1 medium-size yellow bell pepper, chopped
- 1 sweet onion, chopped
- 1/2 teaspoon salt
- 1 1/2 cups fat-free ricotta cheese
- 1 large egg or egg substitute
- 2 cups (8 oz.) shredded part-skim mozzarella cheese, divided
- 1/2 cup freshly grated Parmesan cheese, divided
- 5 cups Marinara sauce, pick your favorite 2 jars, low sodium

- 1 (8-oz.) package no-boil lasagna noodles

Preparation

Preheat oven to 450°. Bake zucchini and mushrooms in a jelly-roll pan coated with cooking spray 12 to 14 minutes or until vegetables are crisp-tender, stirring halfway through. Repeat procedure with bell peppers and onion. Reduce oven temperature to 350°. Toss together vegetables, minced garlic and salt in a bowl.

Stir together ricotta, egg, 1 1/2 cups shredded mozzarella cheese, and 1/4 cup grated Parmesan cheese. In a 13- x 9-inch baking dish coated with cooking spray, spread evenly 1 cup of marinara sauce. Top with 3 noodles, 1 cup sauce, one-third of ricotta mixture, and one-third of vegetable mixture; repeat layers twice, beginning with 3 noodles. Top with remaining noodles and 1 cup sauce. Sprinkle with remaining 1/2 cup shredded mozzarella and 1/4 cup grated Parmesan.

Bake covered at 350° for 45 minutes. Uncover and bake 10 to 15 more minutes or until cheese is melted and golden. Let stand 10 minutes before serving.

Grilled Chicken and Artichoke Salad

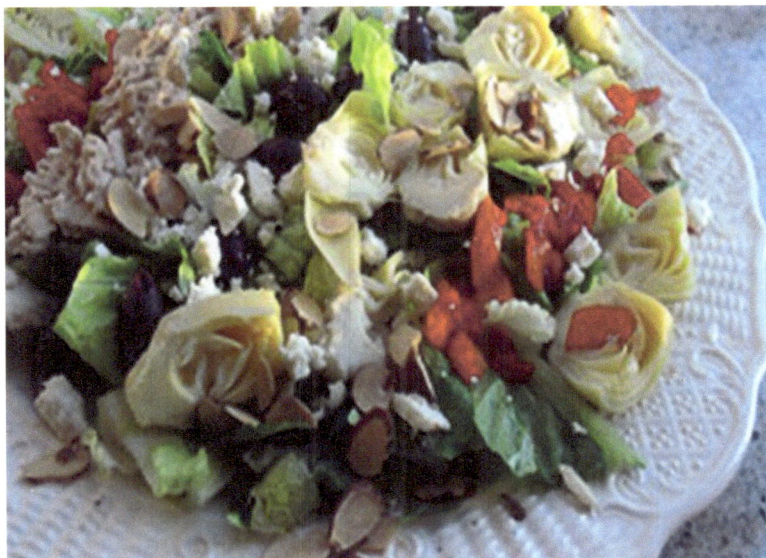

Grilled Chicken and Artichoke Salad

Ingredients:

- 2 grilled skinless chicken breast, found in frozen section, thawed
- 1 bag salad greens
- 1 can artichokes, drained and quartered
- 1 tomato chopped
- 1 small can, sliced black olives drained
- 1/8 cup almond slivers
- 2 oz feta cheese crumbles

Preparation

Warm grilled chicken breast either in oven at 350 degrees for 12 minutes or in microwave for 90 seconds. Chop breast into 1 inch squares. Place all ingredients into a bowl and toss. Serve with your favorite low fat salad dressing.

Clam Fettuccine

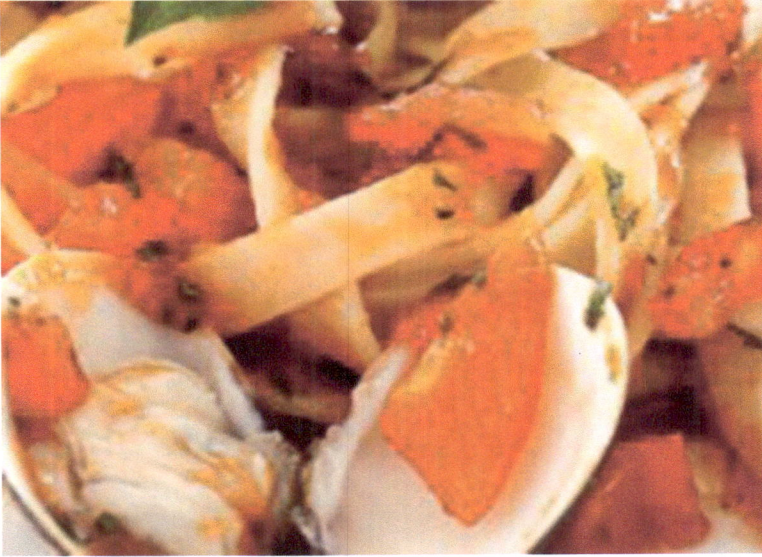

Clam Fettuccine

Ingredients:

- 1 - 16oz package fettuccine pasta

- 2 tablespoons minced garlic

- 2 large tomatoes, seeded and chopped

- 2 cups frozen corn

- 1/2 cup Chardonnay wine

- 1 tablespoon olive oil

- 4 tablespoons chopped fresh basil

- 2 dozen clams in shell or 2 cans (4 ounces each) clams, drained

- 1/4 teaspoon salt

- Ground black pepper, to taste

Preparation

Cook the pasta according to the package preparation. Drain the pasta thoroughly.

In a large saucepan, add the garlic, tomatoes, corn, wine, olive oil and basil. Cover and bring to a boil for 3-5 minutes, stirring frequently. Reduce heat to lowest setting and add the clams and pasta. Toss gently to coat. Season with salt and pepper and it's ready to serve.

Seared Tuna Steak Crusted with Black & White Sesame with Asparagus Spears

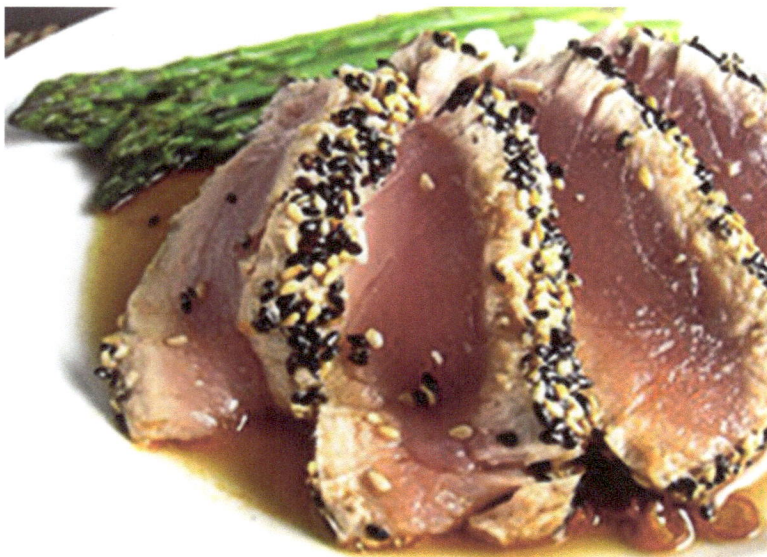

Seared Tuna Steak Crusted with Black & White Sesame with Asparagus Spears

Ingredients:

- 4 Tuna Steaks

- 4 Tablespoons olive oil or canola oil

- 1/2 cup white sesame seed

- 1/4 cup black sesame seed

- Sea salt & course ground black pepper to taste

- Garlic powder to taste

- Cayenne pepper to taste (optional)

- 1 pound asparagus spears

Preparation

Asparagus

Roll asparagus spears in oil and then season with sea salt and garlic powder. Place flat on a cookie sheet. Using aluminum foil to cover the cookie sheet works well for easy clean up.

Place under oven broiler set at 425 degrees and cook until just slight browning appears and then take out and turn spears and cook for one more minute.

Tuna

In a bowl mix the black & white sesame seeds. Season the tuna with your desired combination and roll in the sesame seeds coating the tuna. Use a non stick pan and warm the oil until smoking then place the tuna steaks in the pan and cook until the white sesame seeds start to turn golden, approximately one minute. Flip the tuna over and cook around another minute. Move the tuna steaks to a cutting board and cut into 1/4 inch thick slices and serve with a side of asparagus spears.

Eggplant Parmesan

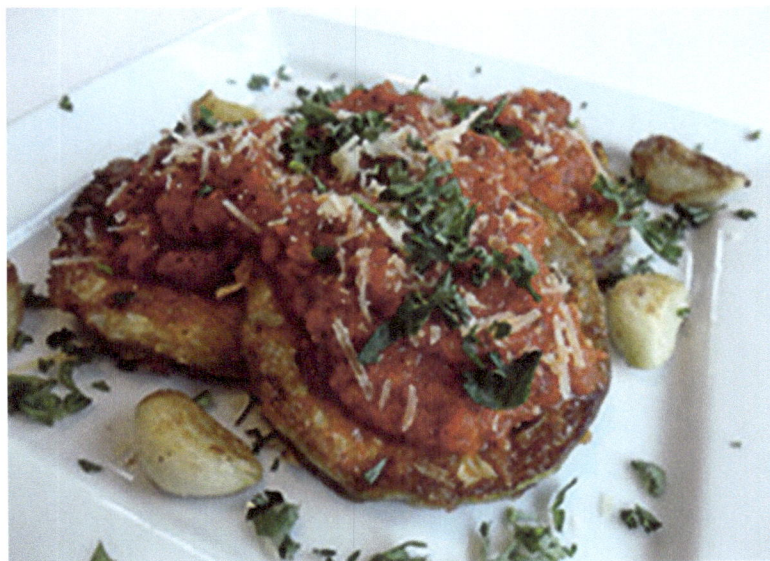

Eggplant Parmesan

Ingredients:

- 2 medium sized eggplants cut crosswise into rounds about 1/3 inch each.

- 2 1/4 teaspoons salt

- 1 Jar of spaghetti sauce 24 oz

- 1 1/2 cups olive oil

- 20 fresh basil leaves torn in half

- 3/4 teaspoon black pepper

- 1/4 teaspoon cayenne pepper (optional)

- 1 cup all-purpose flour

- 5 eggs

- 3 1/2 cup panko Japanese bread crumbs

- 2/3 cup of parmesan cheese finely grated

- 1 lb chilled fresh mozzarella cheese thinly sliced

Preparation

Toss eggplant with 2 teaspoons salt in a colander set over a bowl, then let drain 30 minutes. Preheat oven to 375°F. Mix together flour, 1/4 teaspoon salt, and 1/4 teaspoon pepper in a shallow dish. Beat eggs in a bowl, then stir together panko and 1/3 cup parmesan cheese in a third dish. Doing one slice at a time cover eggplant in flour, shaking off excess, then dip in egg mixer letting excess drip off, and cover in panko until coated. Place the eggplant slices onto sheets of wax paper arranging slices in one layer.

Heat remaining 1 1/2 cups oil in a deep 12-inch nonstick skillet over moderately high heat until hot, then fry eggplant slices turning over once until golden brown 5 to 6 minutes. Then let drain onto paper towels.

Pour 1 cup tomato sauce in bottom of a rectangular 3 1/2-quart 12 x 12 baking dish and spread evenly. Place about one third of eggplant slices in one layer over sauce overlapping slightly if necessary. Cover eggplant with about one third of remaining sauce and one third of mozzarella. Continue layering with remaining eggplant, sauce, and mozzarella. Sprinkle top with remaining 1/3 cup parmesan cheese. Bake uncovered until cheese is melted and golden, and the sauce is bubbling approximately 35 to 40 minutes.

Cajun Black-eyed Peas

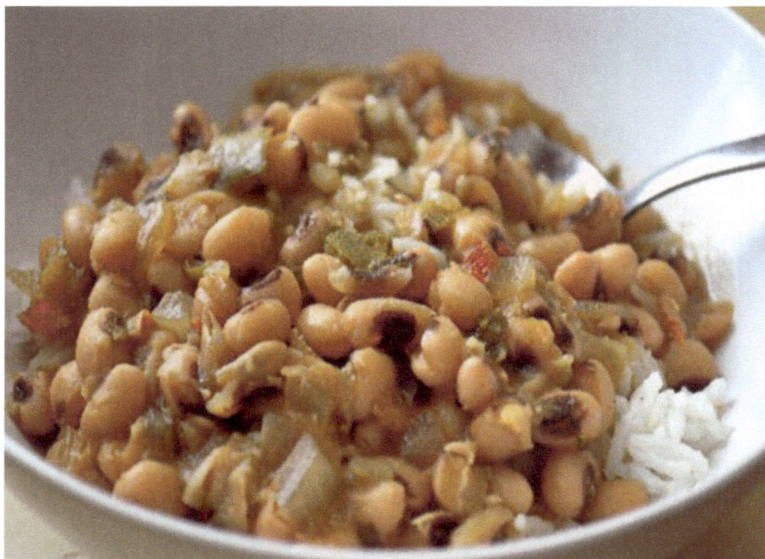

Cajun Black-eyed Peas

Ingredients:

- 3 cups water
- 2 cups dried black-eyed peas
- 1 teaspoon low-sodium chicken-flavored bouillon granules
- 1 15oz can unsalted crushed tomatoes
- 1 large onion finely chopped
- 2 celery stalks finely chopped
- 3 teaspoons minced garlic
- 1/2 teaspoon dry mustard
- 1/4 teaspoon ground ginger
- 1/4 teaspoon cayenne pepper
- 1 bay leaf

Preparation

In a medium saucepan over high heat add 2 cups of the water and black-eyed peas. Bring to a boil for 2 minutes then cover and remove from heat, let stand for 1 hour.

Drain the water leaving the peas in the saucepan. Add the remaining 1 cup of water with the remaining ingredients. Stir together and bring to a boil. Cover and reduce heat to a simmer and cook for 2 hours, stirring occasionally. Add water as necessary to keep the peas covered with liquid.

Remove the bay leaf, then can be served as is or over cooked white rice.

Grilled Salmon with Fresh Herbs

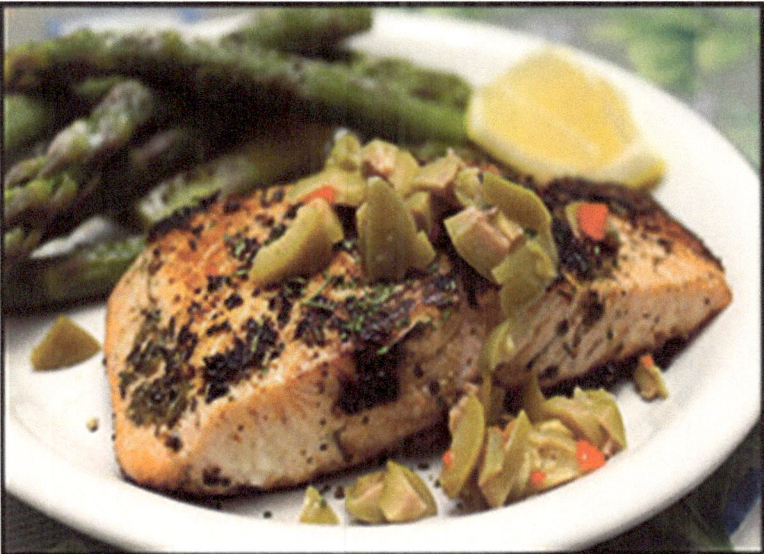

Grilled Salmon with Fresh Herbs

Ingredients:

- 3 tablespoons chopped fresh basil

- 1 tablespoon chopped fresh parsley

- 1 tablespoon minced garlic

- 2 tablespoons lemon juice

- 4 salmon fillets

- Cracked black pepper, to taste

- 4 green olives, chopped

- 4 thin slices lemon

Preparation

Salmon may be prepared on an outdoor grill or inside oven broiler. Preheat either one. Coat the grill rack or broiler pan with cooking spray. In a bowl combine the basil, parsley, minced garlic and lemon juice. Spray the fish with cooking spray. Sprinkle with black pepper. Top each fillet with equal amounts of the basil-garlic mixture.

Place the fish herb-side down on the grill, side up for the oven broiler. Cook over high heat. When the edges turn white in about 3 to 4 minutes, turn the fish over and place on aluminum foil. Move the fish to a cooler part of the grill or reduce the heat. Cook until the fish is opaque throughout when tested with the tip of a knife. Remove salmon and garnish plates with green olives and lemon slices.

Desserts

Peach Crisp

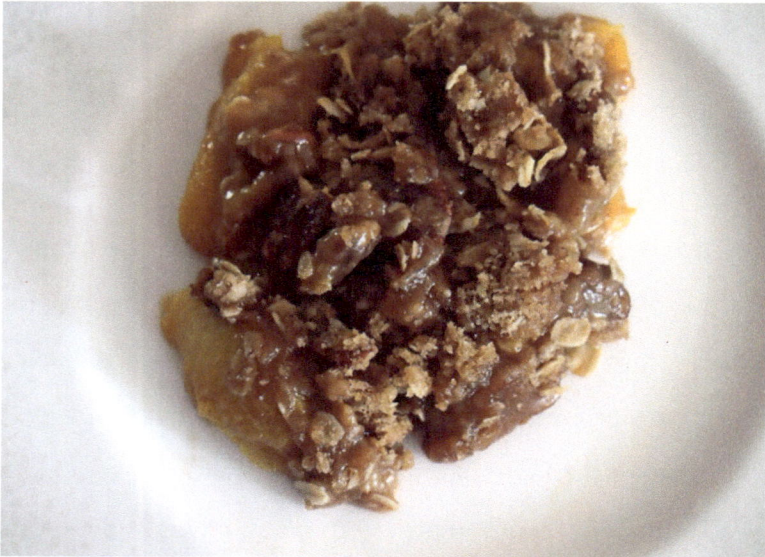

Peach Crisp

Ingredients:

- 8 fresh peaches, peeled, pitted and sliced
- 1 tablespoon lemon juice
- 1/3 teaspoon ground cinnamon
- 1/4 teaspoon ground nutmeg
- 1/2 cup whole-wheat flour
- 1/4 cup brown sugar
- 2 tablespoons trans-free margarine, cut into thin slices
- 1/4 cup quick oats

Preparation

Preheat the oven to 375 F. Lightly coat a 9-inch pie pan with cooking spray.

Arrange peach slices in the pie pan. Sprinkle with lemon juice, cinnamon and nutmeg.

In a bowl mix together flour and brown sugar. Using your hands crumble the margarine into the flour and sugar mixture. Add the oats and mix evenly. Sprinkle the flour mixture on top of the peaches.

Bake until peaches are soft and the topping is browned around 30 minutes, best served warm.

Bananas with Rum Raisin Sauce

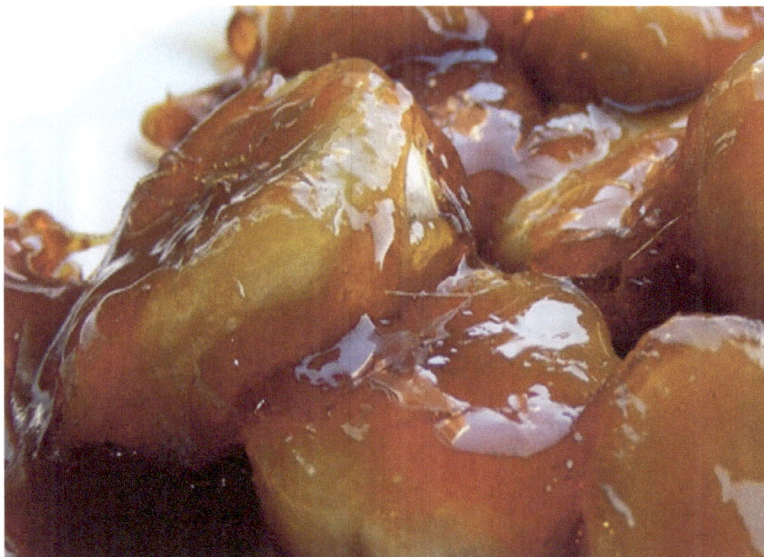

Bananas with Rum Raisin Sauce

Ingredients:

- 1 tablespoon butter

- 1 tablespoon canola oil

- 1 tablespoon honey

- 2 tablespoons brown sugar

- 3 tablespoons low-fat milk

- 1 tablespoon raisins

- 4 bananas

- 2 tablespoons dark rum or apple cider

Preparation

In a small saucepan melt the butter over medium heat. Whisk in canola oil, honey and brown sugar. Stir continuously until brown sugar is dissolved. Stir in milk a little at a time and then cook until the sauce thickens a bit, stir continuously. Remove from the heat and stir in the raisins. Set aside and keep warm.

Peel the bananas, and then cut each crosswise into 3 sections. Cut each section in half lengthwise. Lightly coat a large nonstick frying pan with the canola oil and place over medium-high heat. Add bananas and sauté until they begin to brown. Transfer to a plate.

Add the rum to the pan, bring to a boil and deglaze the pan, stirring constantly cook until rum is reduced by half, approximately 30 to 45 seconds. Return the bananas to the pan to reheat.

Place bananas on serving dishes and drizzle with the warm sauce and serve immediately.

Poached Pears

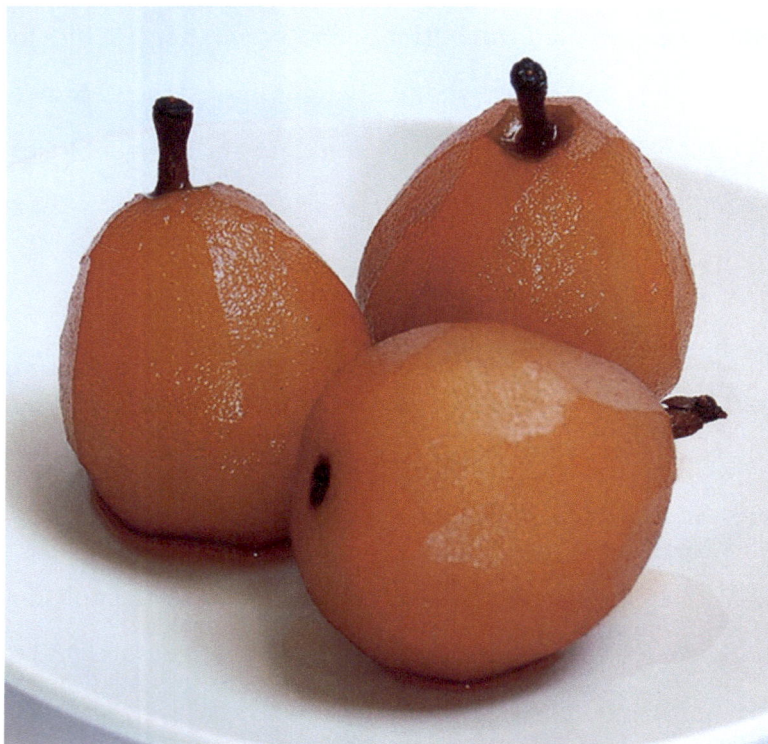

Poached Pears

Ingredients:

- 1 cup orange juice

- 1/4 cup apple juice

- 1 teaspoon ground cinnamon

- 1 teaspoon ground nutmeg

- 4 whole pears

- 1/2 cup fresh raspberries

- 4 fresh mint leaves

Preparation

In a bowl combine the juices, cinnamon and nutmeg. Stir to mix evenly.

Peel the pears and leave the stems. Remove the core from the bottom of the pear. Place in a shallow pan. Add the juice mixture to the pan and set over medium heat. Simmer for about 30 minutes turning pears frequently. Don't boil.

Transfer the pears to individual serving plates. Garnish with raspberries and mint leaves, serve while warm.

More Healthy Eating Tips

Kay Hersom has also written Healthy Heart Diet which is a great complementary book for the Diabetic Diet Plan, and is loaded with additional information that goes "hand in glove" with eating healthy for a diabetic.

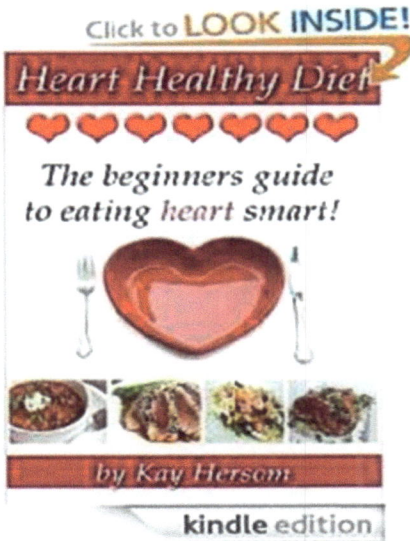

Heart Healthy Diet

Enjoyed the Book?

Thank you for buying this book, I was hoping you could help your fellow book enthusiasts out and when you have a free second leave you honest feedback about this book on Amazon. I certainly want to thank you in advance for doing this.

www.ingramcontent.com/pod-product-compliance
Lightning Source LLC
Chambersburg PA
CBHW041214270326
41930CB00001B/14